JUICING RECIPES FOR WEIGHT LOSS, VITALITY AND HEALTH

By

Ginger Langley

Printed in the United States of America
First Printing: April 2014

ISBN-13: 978-1497557901
ISBN-10: 1497557909

Contents

Introduction

Juicing Recipes for Weight Loss, Vitality and Health are recipes you can create at home in less than five minutes. Choose fresh or frozen fruits and vegetables targeted to specific health conditions.

So much has been written and talked about in the media advising children, teens, and adults to actively seek a healthier lifestyle and to lose weight, that sometimes I think we become selective listeners—we tend to ignore all the advice and warnings unless we have a disease or ailment that needs fixing. But just because you can buy an already-prepared juice at your local store or restaurant doesn't assure you of improved health. In fact, I know many people who never read labels unless they're looking at the calorie count or sodium amount.

This book was written to bring you eight juice recipes that are all targeted to specific areas of your health and body. Short chapters are provided to give you background information and advice regarding specific ailments. You will learn how you can make healthy changes in your life by investing only five minutes a day with JUICING RECIPES and minimal preparation.

For your convenience, I've listed all the juice recipes in one section at the end of the book. For me, I'm not someone who likes reading lots of pages before I get to the recipes. So, I've implemented my personal philosophy for how this book's contents were assembled.

Eight crucial-to-your-health juicing recipes give you an immediate selection of juices that you can make right now in your own kitchen. Juicing for health is not just about tossing some fruits and vegetables into a blender and calling it good. The secret is knowing which vegetable and fruit combinations are targeted to specific health remedies.

For me, I don't need hundreds of recipes. Just give me the ones that taste good and will keep me healthy. I also don't want to have to order special ingredients to make my healthy juices. Maybe you feel the same way. I just want to go to one of my local grocery stores or maybe even a farmer's market in the summer and buy the ingredients I need.

My goal is that after you read this book and try the recipes that you will know which combinations of fruits and vegetables are beneficial to your health. And seriously, I prepare all eight juices every week, and sometimes several a week if my health concerns merit it. These are all my favorite juicing recipes, and I'm hoping they'll become your favorites, too.

About the Author: I am a lifelong lover of healthy foods, and I have a passion for learning more about how I can improve my health and feel more energized. I'm probably no different than others when it comes to going to the doctor. I go for regular checkups and I'm always pleased when the results come back saying that I have no major illness or disease. But life for me wasn't always that way. It seems as the years have gone by, my metabolism has changed, my energy levels have dropped, and I'm not sure I really want to swallow some pharmaceutical company's vitamin supplements without knowing exactly what's in them that they're not telling me about.

The element that I have found most confusing in our medical world is that in most cases, we're not told to seek a nutritionist who can draw up a menu plan for us based on what's happening with the diseases that are taking over our bodies. We're handed a prescription and told to follow up in a certain amount of time to have more tests taken.

This book, then, is my army of juicing recipes that keeps me alive and healthy!

Benefits of Juicing For Beginners

The quality of your life can be greatly affected by the foods that sustain you. A path to a more energetic healthier disease-free lifestyle starts with a diet that is rich in natural foods like fruits and vegetables. Fresh juices can provide the carbohydrates, proteins, and essential fatty acids along with minerals and vitamins that are important factors for your health.

The advantages of a strengthened immune system, increased energy, stronger bones, and a reduced risk of disease are all attainable when you drink fresh juices. Juicing helps provide a nutrient advantage from plant-based foods in a concentrated easily absorbed form for your body.

Juicing for beginners can be quite easy to do, and it is extremely simple to incorporate into your lifestyle. When you find the juicing machine or high-powered blender that is right for you, you can start experimenting with different combinations of fruits and vegetables to find the taste that you like most.

There are many juicers on the market today and you need to pick from the wide variety that is available to you. The function of a juicer is to actually separate the liquid from the pulp. Fiber is important but the juice is what nourishes us. A blender can liquefy and chop up produce at high speeds, but it does not separate the juice from the pulp.

It is very important to follow the instructions of your juicer's or blender's manual before you start to use it. Although it may seem pretty simple and obvious, please take the time to read through your manual or watch an instructional video if it is included with your machine. This will help you get the most benefit in the shortest amount of time.

The most important thing to think about when looking for a juice machine is to make sure that you find something that will clean easily. If the juicer is difficult to use, you are more likely not to use it, and it will just sit on your counter.

It is important when you start to use your juicer that you use only organic vegetables and produce. Wash everything thoroughly. This is important because you do not want any chemicals or pesticides in your juice. There are many juicing-for-beginners recipes available in books, video, and on the web to help get you started.

The list of benefits of juicing for beginners goes on and on. The key benefit of consuming fresh juices is that it can provide your body with a higher level of antioxidants, which in turn can help protect your body against many ailments, such as heart disease, cancer, and other degenerative conditions.

Power Juicing in Only 5 Minutes a Day

Do you have an active lifestyle? If you often feel tired or do not have enough energy to go through your daily routine, you should give power juicing a chance. Preparing some delicious and healthy juices will help you get more vitamins into your body and give you plenty of energy.

Power juicing is an excellent way to get your five daily portions of fruits and vegetables. A lot of individuals do not get enough fruits and vegetables in their diet, because they do not have time to cook or do not enjoy these foods. You can easily prepare one glass of juice for your breakfast and your dinner.

You can prepare healthy juices rich in vitamins by mixing different ingredients. Experiment and you will eventually find juices you really love. It is best to use a small number of ingredients and add an apple or another fruit to mask the strong taste of some vegetables. Avoid using more than three or four ingredients for a more enjoyable taste.

Choose ingredients rich in vitamins to get the energy you need. Each glass of juice should include one or two vegetables, such as broccoli, dark leafy greens, carrots, spinach, or kale. These vegetables are rich in vitamins A, B C and K.

If you need to sweeten the taste of the vegetables, an apple, a pear, or a lemon is a great choice. You should also add some strawberries, raspberries, pineapple, mango, kiwi, banana, or passion fruit for more vitamins A, B and C. You might be tempted to only mix fruits to make a sweet drink, but juicing is healthier if you add at least one vegetable to each glass of juice. Vegetables are rich in vitamins and do not contain as much sugar as fruits do.

Power juicing is very easy and will help you live and feel more dynamic in everything you do.

Start experimenting today with your favorite fruits and vegetables by choosing a recipe from this book.

What You Should Know Before Buying a Juicer or Blender

If you have made the decision to enter into a healthier lifestyle, then you need to buy a juicer or blender in order to help you realize your goals. Today there are many incredible options that you can choose from. You simply must take your needs into account and then search for your options that are within your budget. Before you know it, you can be enjoying juice and reaping all of the benefits that come along with a healthier diet.

If you do not want to spend too much money on a piece of equipment that is going to just sit on your counter collecting dust, take the time to look in to all of the features that you can choose from. Consider your reasoning behind your quest to buy a juicer or blender, and you will be able to pick and choose one that fulfills all of your needs. When you can understand the differences between each juicer versus a blender,

11

then you will be able to make an informed decision on buying the right one for your household.

Take notice of the price ranges for juicers and blenders. You can look at spending anywhere from $40 upwards to more than $750, depending on the type of device that sparks your interest. The cheaper models are great for someone who is going to partake in casual juicing, maybe once per day or even every other day. These less expensive models can work less effectively or even break with excessive use.

For the person who is going to be juicing several times per day and pretty much every day of the week, it might be important to buy a juicer or high-speed blender like a Vitamix that has the capacity to stand up to such wear and use. Some of these larger models are not only meant to be used daily, but they can often make large batches of juice at a time. The more juice per pound you need, the more you will usually spend when you buy a juicer.

Finally, it is extremely important that you look at a number of customer reviews on the type of juicer that has caught your eye. Listening to what users have to say and finding out the recipes that work best with certain models will help you to make an informed decision prior to your purchase. When you are ready to buy a juicer or blender, all of the information you've acquired will help you successfully choose just the right machine for your needs and lifestyle.

Reap the Benefits of a Green Juice Smoothie

If you are new to the world of juicing, chances are you have not heard about green juices and their many benefits. However, once you start to research juicing and all of the different juice combinations that are out there, you are bound to find out all about green juice options along with green juice smoothie recipes that will give your mind, body, and soul an incredible health boost. When you are ready to get juicing, simply look up a little bit more about your options and you can dive in.

Many people have multiple recipes for green juice. Most of the common combinations used today include ingredients such as celery and cucumber with the addition of other green veggies or fruits such as spinach, cilantro, sprouts, lime, zucchini, or even parsley.

Picking and choosing the ingredients that you like best will often yield a result that is quite flavorful. Once you come up with a good combination, you can add other things into your green juice smoothie to bring up the levels of vitamins and minerals.

As with other varieties of juices for health and wellness, a green juice smoothie is a great way to help boost your mood as well as your energy level. Many juicing fanatics will look forward to drinking their smoothie first thing in the morning to get them going and energized for whatever their day will bring their way. As a matter of fact, many nutritionists will even tell you that a properly formulated green juice smoothie can help to eliminate the need for prescriptions and medications for anxiety or mood.

Certainly, when you are taking in a decent amount of green fruits and veggies, you will see a difference in your bodily functions. Many people who are juice drinkers will find that they are more regular with a marked improvement in overall bowel health. This is why a lot of people who are battling irregularity will add more fibrous green vegetables to their diet. When you drink a green juice smoothie, you are able to get these foods easily in one drink.

No matter what your reasoning might be for trying a green juice smoothie, you are bound to find yourself addicted to the results. Once you start feeling good on the inside, it will start to show through on the outside and permeate throughout your daily interactions. Finding the perfect green juice smoothie is easy as long as you are open to the various ingredients that you have to choose from.

How Juicing Software Can Help Your Juice Diet

Juice is a wonderfully healthy drink that can provide your body with vitamins, minerals, complex carbohydrates, essential fatty acids, and even protein. Fresh juice contains natural enzymes and pigments like flavonoids, chlorophyll, and carotenes. Today, a juice diet can be simpler and healthier because of juicing software that is now available.

For instance, which juices taste best when combined together? What are the health benefits of all the various fruits and vegetables? Are there juices that are curative for specific health problems? All of these are questions that can be simply answered using your new juicing software.

Many programs will even set up a daily menu to ensure you are getting the healthiest benefits of the juices that you drink, and that you're rotating your fruits and vegetables.

Juicing software can help you choose specific vegetables and fruits and outline for you the nutritional advantages of each. Also, you will learn how diets with a large percentage of uncooked fruits and vegetables can aid you in losing weight. It is a great way to control both your blood pressure and your blood sugar levels.

You will find that eating fruits and vegetables raw is very filling. Cooking reduces over 90 percent of the water-soluble vitamins such as K, E, D and A. Because uncooked fruits and vegetables are more nutrient-dense, they are much more satisfying to your body—and therefore more filling. Your juicing software will give you the right combination of fruits and vegetables to keep your metabolism running efficiently and your weight loss on target.

Juicing is a great way to get your body's digestive system kick-started. It allows quick absorption of nutrient-dense foods that will increase your energy, which is one of the real advantages of losing weight through proper nutrition. Fresh juices, as part of a well-balanced diet, will provide you with the necessary energy to burn calories and fat and provide you with the necessary fuel for exercise.

Another thing you will learn with your new juicing software is how to increase your daily fiber intake with specific juices. Fiber-rich fruits and vegetables are important to your health and well-being.

Using your new juicing software to plan your daily selections will enhance your well-balanced diet while adding flavor and zest. It will give you some tasty recipes while helping you understand the basics of nutrition. Why not start adding the advantages of healthy juices to your diet?

Easy Juicing For Weight Loss

Whenever the Spring season approaches, we are naturally looking to possibly lose some weight. That's when we'll think about doing a detox so we can get extra healthy by getting rid of all those toxins and feeling that vibrant energy again. It's no wonder that the media has gone overboard about juicing for weight loss right now.

Juicing is without doubt really good for your body. You can do juicing in various ways. In any case, it is a wonderful way to consume copious amounts of fresh raw fruit and veggies, and your body will thank you for it.

There are a lot of people who believe that you should only eat fruit on an empty stomach and that ideally fruit and fruit juice should be consumed in the morning. Well, fruit, without a doubt, is a wonderful way to detoxify and cleanse your body. Of course, the best choice would be to consume locally grown and organic ingredients.

You can also enjoy a mix of fruit and vegetables. Kale is very popular, because its dark green leaves are full of nutrients. The same could be said of spinach. Kale or spinach combined with a green apple or two and maybe some celery is a great drink. Some vegetables have more water content than others. Cucumbers, for example, are great combined with other veggies in a juice.

With juicing, you can follow recipes or create your own. Just make sure you enjoy a good variety of fruits and vegetables and preferably those in season. With a good juicer or blender, you can basically juice anything.

The reason for juicing for weight loss is that the nutrients your body receives from the fruit and vegetables will fill you up. Weight loss is hard when you eat processed and fast foods, because although you are full, soon your body is craving food again, simply because you have virtually been eating "dead food" that your body has a hard time coping with, and it eventually ends up expanding your fat cells. Juicing enables your body to replenish itself. You will feel good, your skin will glow, and your body will not crave extra food. Plus, you might even be able to get rid of those prescription drugs when your health improves.

If you are serious about juicing, then check out the slow juicers. You can easily do some research on the internet but basically these slow juicers are popular because not only do they produce more juice than the average juicer, but the juice has a higher percentage of nutrients. They are more expensive but worth it in the end.

Not only is it easy juicing for weight loss, but it works!

Is Juicing For Hair Loss A Good Option?

Have you been losing your hair? Hair loss is often caused by a diet that is poor in vitamins. You can introduce more vitamins in your diet by eating five portions of fruits and vegetables a day. Juicing gives you the opportunity to get your five portions of fruits or vegetables in a glass. Keep reading if you want to learn more about juicing for hair loss.

Juicing is a great way to introduce more fruits and vegetables in your diet if you do not have much time to cook. You can easily prepare a glass of juice in a few minutes if you have all the ingredients you need at home. Look for fruits and vegetables rich in vitamins A, B and C for stronger hair.

You should invest in a quality juicer. There are several types of juicers to choose from and you should try finding one that corresponds to your needs. Juicing for hair loss is a good solution but you need to be consistent with it. Choose a juicer that is very easy to use and clean so you can have a glass of juice a day.

Create your own juices. You can find vitamin A in sweet potatoes, carrots, dark leafy greens, butternut squash, cantaloupe, and apricots. Combine these different ingredients and add an apple or a pear to mask the strong taste of dark leafy greens or of another vegetable you do not enjoy.

If you need more vitamin B in your diet, make juices with asparagus, artichokes, broccoli, Brussels sprouts, or pumpkin. You can also add some avocado, blackberries, orange, papaya, passion fruit, raspberries, or strawberries. Try mixing two or three of these ingredients to find a flavor you like.

You can create a juice rich in vitamin C by mixing some broccoli, butternut squash, green peppers, Brussels sprout or some grapefruit, guava, kiwi, lychee, mango, pineapple or strawberries. It is usually best to mix three ingredients and add an apple or a similar fruit if you do not enjoy the strong taste of the vegetables you used.

Juicing for hair loss is very efficient if you use your juicer once a day and create healthy juices rich in vitamins. Experiment with different ingredients until you find recipes you really like. It is usually best to mix a small number of ingredients and always add a fruit for a sweeter taste.

Juicing for Arthritis Works

More and more people suffer from arthritis and even children can nowadays get the disease. There are many who believe that arthritis is caused by the body being too acidic. This is something we should all be aware of. If you drink a cup of coffee, for example (and who doesn't?), your body becomes acidic. The easy solution to this is to drink a large glass of water afterwards. Processed foods, fast foods, and commercial sodas are acidic forming. Today, we are eating and drinking more and more acidic-forming foods and drinks.

We can help our bodies become more alkaline by consuming more fresh fruits and vegetables as well as drinking more quality water. Stay away from sugars and white flour as well as the above mentioned foods if you have arthritis. Also, it could be that nightshade plants like tomatoes and zucchinis are also not good for people with arthritis.

So how do we easily consume more fresh fruit and veggies? Juicing makes it an easy fix and juicing for arthritis works wonders. If you don't yet have a juicer, a slow juicer is the way to go. If you have a juicer, then you just need to purchase some produce. Juicing for arthritis works best in the morning. Make it your new breakfast regime.

On the next page are several juicing recipes that will help with your arthritis.

Papaya and Blueberry Juice

You just need a quarter of a freshly peeled papaya and up to two cups of fresh blueberries for a great tasting drink.

Carrot and Broccoli Juice

You need the orange parts of three medium carrots, one apple without the core, half a lemon without the peel and half a cup of fresh broccoli pieces. This is a wonderful tonic.

Carrot and Celery Juice with Pineapple

The pineapple and lemon in this juice give it a nice kick. You will require one teaspoon of lemon juice, four ounces of pineapple, five carrots, and two celery stalks.

Remember when you drink these delicious concoctions that you should sip slowly. There are a lot of fruits and vegetables in the juices and it's like eating a meal, so take your time. A good way is to have your fresh juice with you all morning and take a sip or two when you feel like it.

Juicing for arthritis works and is a powerful way to alleviate the pain and inflammation this disease causes.

Juicing For Diabetes Is a Wonderful Solution

When managing your diabetes, it's so important that you're eating the right foods and watching your glucose level. With so many manufactured foods for sale with high levels of sugar and carbohydrates, how can you win?

One great thing you can do to monitor your blood sugar and eat the right foods containing vitamins and nutrients that your body needs is to pursue juicing for diabetes. You see, your body needs the right type of natural sweeteners that fruit can provide. Not only that, but you need to be eating plenty of fresh foods that come in the form of fruits and vegetables when you're eating your balanced diet. Third, juicing for diabetes allows you to promote metabolism and digestion thanks to the liquidity and of course the vitamins and nutrients that you're consuming.

Think about the great effects! I have been juicing for quite some time, and I have also been able to keep my weight down. If you have diabetes, then you are aware that being overweight only complicates things. Juicing for diabetes is a way to keep your weight under control.

I like to juice all kinds of different smoothies, and I have been learning all the different combinations. There are other things you can add to the fruits and vegetables as well to help get what you need. It's like a meal in a glass!

I have been telling my friends about it as well. I am part of a diabetes support group, and I recently told all of them about my juicing experiences. Now, guess what we do once a week? We have a juicing party on Fridays, and everyone comes together to enjoy smoothies and learn about how juicing can impact their lives. It's really a great experience, and we all have a lot of fun doing it.

Why don't you continue to take a further look at how juicing can help you with your diabetes? You are going to be amazed at what you find out. Surely, you are going to realize that you definitely want to take advantage of this wonderful solution for you to manage your diabetes much better.

Reasons for Juicing for Allergies

Juicing is renowned for its healing properties. Many people choose it for weight loss as well. So let's get our juicers and blenders out and consider juicing for allergies. *With the right recipes, you can help rid your body of, and even prevent, allergies.

One reason for juicing is that juicing separates the liquids from the pulp and seeds in the fruits and vegetables used. This resulting juice releases vitamins and minerals that help the body to heal and recover from allergies and other conditions.

Many people swear by using a lemonade-parsley juice drink to eliminate allergies. Here is what they use. Shred or tear two small cups of parsley, chop up a cucumber and peel two lemons. Now slice up a green apple and add in a two-inch knob of fresh ginger. Put this through your juicer. If it's a bit tart, add some honey or agave to taste. You may need to add a bit of filtered water to this if it's too strong. Drink it down and do this daily until you achieve results by reduced allergy symptoms. Hint: If using honey, use local honey; it will provide better immunity to allergies if you choose local.

Another reason for juicing is that juicing is nature's best medicine. It provides the body with detoxifying elements that help us to flush the toxins out of our systems and adds necessary vitamins and minerals to our bodies. Many people don't have time to grab a healthy breakfast, but by juicing, you can still get the benefits you need for a healthy immune system that is allergy free.

An important reason for juicing is that vitamins are enhanced when fruits and vegetables are juiced. Using local foods and local honey helps eliminate the allergens even faster. Local foods and honey are those that are grown nearby.

Next time you think about a morning latte, think about the benefits of juicing for allergies instead. Your body will take in the required nutrients and vitamins to fight off your allergies in lieu of all that caffeine, which will leave you feeling flat and lifeless in a few short hours.

Consider a spicy kick when juicing for allergies. Your body may benefit from an addition of garlic, cayenne, or ginger and open your sinus congestion right up. Just a small addition of any of these will help to reduce congestion and swelling. Also, the other flavors can help to cover up the potent flavor if you don't care for it.

Juicing is nature's best medicine.

JUICING RECIPES:
BETTER HEALTH IN JUST FIVE MINUTES

This section of the book contains the eight healthy-life recipes that I have created to maximize the health benefits you can achieve by spending five minutes a day making nutritious juice combinations with fruits and vegetables. Enjoy!

In case you're wondering why I spell out all my ingredients rather than using numbers or abbreviations, it's because when I would write recipes on cards for friends or family members, sometimes all the abbreviations made the recipe turn out wrong...imagine measuring one teaspoon of something when I was saying "measure it." And the person making the recipe thought that "it" meant one teaspoon, or worse, since I use capital letters when I print...IT (one tablespoon). Oh my!

My Favorite "Green Juice for Life" Recipe

This juicing recipe contains lots of iron that makes your blood cells healthy and gives you more range of motion and flexibility for your muscles. Besides being good for your blood and your muscles, this delicious green juice provides more Vitamin K than is normally required by any health regime. Vitamin K is known to provide better health for your blood and bones.

Yield: 1 serving

Prep time: 5 minutes

Shopping List to Make This Juice: kale, English cucumber, green grapes, Granny Smith apple

Ingredients:

One cup kale, sliced (or 3 leaves)

One Seedless English Cucumber, sliced thick

One cup green seedless grapes (approximately 25)

One Granny Smith apple (about 4 oz.), cored, not peeled, large chunks

One-half cup water

Directions:

In your blender, add all five ingredients (kale, cucumber, grapes, apple, and water). Blend until the mixture is smooth. If you wish, you can strain the juice by placing a small sieve over your glass before pouring the juice. If the juice is too thick for your preference, then just add a little more water.

Drink immediately or store in the refrigerator for a maximum of two days, making sure you shake the juice before pouring it after it's been refrigerated.

Nutritional Information (Per Serving):

110 calories

0.6g fat

3g protein

27 g carbohydrates

3g fiber

0.0mg cholesterol

1mg iron

19mg sodium

77mg calcium

This is My Go-To "Pink Lady Cherple" Recipe

This scrumptious juice packs more vitamins into just one glass of juice than anyone would imagine, and it makes me instantly feel great and ready to start my day.

I named this juice Pink Lady Cherple, because the color is a light pink that a lady would love, and Cherple is my attempt at making a word out of cherries, pear, and apple.

This powerful juice contains vitamins A, B, C, and E, which means that it has the ability to provide energy and fuel for your body. The combination of vitamins A and C is known to increase the production of collagen, which we all know makes our skin look younger and firmer. This juice is known to fight aging, give you stronger bones (think no osteoporosis), and your skin becomes more radiant.

Yield: 1 serving

Prep time: 5 minutes

Shopping List to Make This Juice: cherries (fresh or frozen), one medium red apple, two ripe pears

Ingredients:

One-half cup cherries (fresh or frozen); just remember to remove the pits, since they don't do well in a blender.

Two ripe medium-sized pears with the cores removed. If you want to weigh them at the store, you'll need about one pound. I like Bartlett pears if they're within my budget when I shop.

One medium red apple (any variety), core removed and chopped into chunks. Leave the skin on if you have a powerful blender.

Directions:

In your blender, add all three ingredients (cherries, pears, apple), and blend until smooth. Add water to make the mixture thinner if you want. Strain for extra pulp or remnant seeds before pouring the juice into a glass.

You can drink it immediately or store it in your fridge for up to two days. Just know that sometimes the color changes if you leave it overnight in your fridge. But if you're going to make it, why not drink it and get a powerful vitamin hit to start your day?

Nutritional Information (Per Serving):

192 calories

0.4g fat

1g protein

51g carbs

8g fiber

0.0mg cholesterol

1mg iron

2mg sodium

29mg calcium

Purple Royalty Reigns Recipe

Even though you only have three types of fruit to mix for this dynamic and powerful juice, the berries contain so many antioxidants that the badly invaded cells in your body could possibly run scared when you drink this. Plus, the bonus is that this is another wonderful anti-aging drink that makes you just feel so good.

I call this juice Purple Royalty Reigns, because I usually manage to get purple-blue stains on myself and my kitchen counter if I'm not careful. (You've been warned!)

Yield: 1 serving

Prep time: 5 minutes

Ingredients:

One cup blueberries (fresh or thawed from frozen)

Two cups mango, peeled and cut into chunks

One cup strawberries (fresh or thawed from frozen; cut strawberries in half

One-quarter cup water

Directions:

In your blender, (am I really saying to do this for every recipe?), add the three fruits and the water. Blend until smooth, adding extra water if it's too thick for your liking.

This juice can be refrigerated for up to two days. Just remember to shake it before pouring it into a glass if you've stored it in your fridge.

Nutritional Information (Per Serving):

151 calories per

1g fat

2g protein

38g carbohydrates

5g fiber

0.0mg cholesterol

1mg iron

3mg sodium

27g calcium

I Need a Hydration Boost Recipe

So many of my health dilemmas used to previously be wrapped around the fact that I didn't drink enough water, or else it got leached from my body somehow. That's when my nutritionist told me to start making my own juice so I could get the electrolytes that would keep me hydrated. In this hydration-boost recipe, you'll find natural fruit sugars that instantly bump up your energy levels, and the coconut water provides the electrolytes you'll need to stay hydrated. Who knew?

Yield: 1 serving

Prep time: 5 minutes

Ingredients:

One cup peaches (thawed from frozen), sliced. I usually calculate this at about 8 ounces.

Three-Quarters of a cup of coconut water (nowadays this is available at most grocery stores); if it's not available, you can just use water, but then you won't get the hydration benefit.

One can (20-oz.) of lychees in syrup; drain the syrup off and rinse the lychees. If you live in an area where you can get fresh lychees, then use about 21 of them, making sure that you peel them and remove the seeds.

Directions:

In your blender, add the peaches, coconut water and lychees, and blend until the mixture has a smooth consistency. As with the other juice recipes in this book, you can refrigerate the juice for up to two days.

Nutritional Information (Per Serving):

105 calories
6g fat
2g protein
26g carbs
3g fiber
0.0mg cholesterol
1mg iron
95mg sodium
26mg calcium

The Cold-and-Flu-Chaser Miracle Recipe

This recipe is a variation of one that a friend told me about many years ago when I was constantly suffering from a weak immune system. Before that time, I was always heading to the doctor for vitamin C shots, or else I'd buy Emergen-C by the box, or I'd get a bottle of chewable Vitamin C tablets.

I drink huge quantities of this juice the minute I feel a cold coming on. It just seems to ward off the nasties, like when you get up in the morning and sigh because your throat feels scratchy. And sometimes I just drink it to build my immune system.

Since this juicing recipe contains the miracle kiwi fruit, I will head to my warehouse shopping store like Costco to buy a bag of kiwis for a ridiculously low price for the number of kiwis I get. But if you just want to try this recipe out, you might want to get the kiwis from your local grocery store. But like here where I live, the grocers get crazy and price them like $0.99 each, like they sometimes do with avocados. It depends how stubborn I feel that day whether I'll fork over the dough until I can make a trip to the warehouse store. I know...sometimes I'd probably spend more in gas for my car to drive to the warehouse store than if I would have coughed up three dollars for three kiwis. Anyway, let's get you that recipe.

First, let me just say that kiwis provide almost twice as much Vitamin C that you'll need in any typical day, and they certainly give you more vitamins that other citrus fruits.

Yield: 1 serving

Prep time: 5 minutes

Ingredients:

Three kiwis, approximately 12 total ounces; but who's really weighing them? Peel off the furry skin and cut the fruit into fourths.

One grapefruit, peeled and segmented (**Word of Caution** here: If you're taking thyroid medication, talk to your doctor before eating any type of grapefruit; a time requirement is necessary so the grapefruit doesn't cancel the thyroid medicine's effectiveness).

Two medium oranges, peeled and divided into segments.

Directions:

Place all ingredients into your blender, and blend until smooth. You can strain the juice if you wish, and you can also thin the mixture by adding a little bit of water.

Keeps in your refrigerator for up to two days.

Nutritional Information (Per Serving):

156 calories

1g fat

3g protein

38g carbohydrates

6g fiber

0.0mg cholesterol

1mg iron

5mg sodium

79mg calcium

Bridge Over Nutty Water Recipe

This recipe is awesome for repairing and building your muscles, whether you've just had surgery or your body is "burning" after you've spent time at the gym working out. This juice also contains more potassium than you'd normally get if you ate two bananas. Plus all that potassium helps to balance your intake of fluids and electrolytes.

Yield: 1 service

Prep time: 5 minutes

Ingredients:

One medium red apple, cored and diced

One-quarter cup whole, raw almonds

Two medium oranges, peeled and divided into segments

One small sweet potato (not yams); scrub the skin well and chop into big chunks

One-half cup water

Directions:

Place all the ingredients into your blender and blend until smooth. Strain the juice using a small wire handheld strainer over the drinking glass as you pour in the juice.

Refrigerate for up to two days.

Nutritional Information (Per Serving):

231 calories
9.1g fat
6g protein

36g carbs

7g fiber

0.0mg cholesterol

1mg iron

24g sodium

106mg calcium

The Five-Letter Word Recipe

For some reason, I despise the word "DETOX" (the five-letter word), but this juice is excellent for cleaning out your system of all its ugly things that like to take up residence in your body, even when your digestive system doesn't want them there.

This juicing recipe contains root vegetables that offer high-fiber benefits to your body, and fruit, which makes the river bed slippery so those ugly things can move through your digestive tract at record speed. Finally, to bring some sunshine to this juicing journey through your body, the ginger helps to calm your stomach.

Yield: 1 service

Prep time: 5 minutes

Ingredients:

Two tablespoons fresh ginger, peeled and roughly chopped

One medium-sized red apple, cored and cut into chunks

Four carrots, scrubbed clean and sliced (don't scape the peeling off)

One medium fresh beet, scrubbed and chopped (Beware: Beet juice stains, so this is best done over your sink)

One cup of water

Directions:

Blend all the ingredients in your blender, add water to thin the mixture, and strain the juice. Keeps in the fridge for up to two days.

Nutritional Information (Per Serving):

155 calories

0.7g fat

3g protein

37g carbohydrates

8g fiber

0.0mg cholesterol

1mg iron

168mg sodium

62mg calcium

The Anti-Cancer, Anti-Disease Juice Recipe

Whether you've had cancer before and you're a survivor, or you've had a life-threatening disease, this is one juice recipe that should be on the top of your list for twice-weekly consumption.

Yield: 1 serving

Prep time: 5 minutes

Ingredients:

Two cups of broccoli with their stems on, chopped

Two-third cup of watercress (sold in local grocery stores; if you've never seen it, ask your produce manager)

Three medium carrots, peeled and chopped

Three cauliflower florets, chopped

One red apple, cored and cut in fourths

Five Kale leaves

Directions:

Put all ingredients into your juicer or a high-speed blender like a Vitamix and blend.

Nutritional Information (Per Serving):

64 calories

0.4g total fat

3.5g protein

14g carbohydrates

61mg sodium

3.9g fiber

5828ug beta-carotene

73mg Vitamin C

74mg calcium

0.8mg iron

50ug folate

26mg magnesium

0.4mg zinc

1.4ug selenium

Thank you for buying my book. Now all I ask is that you try the recipes and spend just five minutes a day to achieve better health.

Wishing you all the best,

Ginger Langley

Did You Like This Book?

It looks like you've made it all the way to the end of my book. I'm very happy you enjoyed it enough to get all the way through the recipes and health benefits. Hopefully, you've earmarked several recipes that you'll try today or this week.

If you liked the book, would you be open to leaving me an honest review? If you can take a minute, I'd really appreciate you writing a review on the Amazon website so others can discover how easy and healthy it is to spend five minutes creating a juice that you'll love. It would really mean a lot to me.

Thank you!

Ginger Langley

About the Author

Ginger Langley lives in the Pacific Northwest, and she loves to cook and experiment with new healthy recipes.

Don't forget to check out these best-selling books, also by Ginger Langley:

Coconut Milk Recipes: 21 Quick & Easy Meals for Breakfast, Lunch, Dinner, and Dessert

Juicing Recipes for Weight Loss, Vitality and Health

Organic Homemade Skin Care Recipes for Beginners: Easy and Simple Instructions for Natural Remedies

Vitamin Water Recipes: Quick & Easy Homemade Vitamin Drinks Made From Fruits & Vegetables

Contact Me

If you have any questions for me, or if you have a story you'd like to share about how juicing improved your well-being, you can contact me here:

gingerlangley1@gmail.com

NOTES